NAKED UNDER MY COAT

WRITING UNDER THE INFLUENCE OF PARKINSON'S

Jocelyn Burgener

Produced by:

FriesenPress
Suite 300 – 852 Fort Street
Victoria, BC, Canada V8W 1H8

www.friesenpress.com

www.jocelynburgener.ca

Distributed to the trade by The Ingram Book Company

TABLE OF CONTENTS

FEARFUL

HEARTFELT

Jocelyn Burgener

NAKED UNDER MY COAT: **REVIEWS**

"Skillfully switches between prose and poetry."

Naked Under My Coat! is brimming with life: It has energy, rhythms, eccentricities, happiness, sadness and beauty!" Frances Wright, Famous 5 Founding Chair. Readers will quickly become the BFF of this book. The story-telling style is refreshing and skillfully switches between prose and poetry.

I loved the intimate feeling which Jocelyn created, and was sad when the story ended. Here's to the next book. Tell us even more about this fascinating writer and how she copes through her writing. Jocelyn's Famous 5 poem is fabulous! Both visually and literally. The Famous 5 are no doubt shouting, *«Bravo, Jocelyn! You are one of us! Thank you!»*

Frances Wright: Famous 5 Foundation

"The felt-meaning of the words"

In one of her stories in this collection, Jocelyn Burgener writes: "Each encounter revealed a familiarity that was eerie…Perhaps need and fear have an aura of familiarity because they are so tangible." The two sentences are the writer's fingertips pressing the inside of the reader's wrist; the felt-meaning of the words that fill the book. It is a book filled with the courage of someone coming home to a house with an intruder inside, stepping through the burgled door intending not just to survive but to befriend.

Peter Stockland: CARDUS, Senior Director, Publications and Media

"An aura of intimacy."

Jocelyn creates an aura of intimacy in her writing. The reader is invited into the conversation, even as she is picking up the pieces of her life.

Joan Crockatt: MP

"She speaks with clarity."

Naked Under My Coat reveals the author's keen powers of observation. She speaks with clarity whether posing questions, or exposing a painful truth.

Linda Garson: Editor-In-Chief, Culinaire Magazine

"Poignant in their description of truth."

The beauty of Jocelyn Burgener's writing lies in its vulnerability. Her words - in prose or in poetry - are poignant in their description of truth.

Pastor John Van Sloten: New Hope Church

"Naked Under My Coat holds many pleasant and thought-provoking surprises."

Jocelyn Burgener's book of ideas, insights, stories and poetry kept me reading even as my daily newspaper press deadlines closed in on me. That's a good sign. "Naked Under My Coat: Writing Under the Influence of Parkinson's" holds many pleasant and thought-provoking surprises. As a self-described DLHPAC

(Dyslectic, Left-Handed, Parkinson's Afflicted Crocheter) there is something for everyone in Jocelyn's collection of naked exploration of the human condition and autobiography.

Licia Corbella: Editorial Page Editor, Calgary Herald

Jocelyn Burgener

DEDICATION

To my family and the journey we share.

Jocelyn Burgener

INTRODUCTION

Sometime in the late nineteen-nineties I began to write. Tenuously, perceptions became words, then phrases, a concept, a poem. Ideas became conversations, leading to stories. Observations became tangible, and my intention to publish a reality, and so *"Naked Under My Coat"* evolved.

I chose the subtitle *"Writing Under the Influence of Parkinson's"* as the urge to write was coincidental with the onset of my Parkinson's. I consider my Parkinson's a gift.

Rigidity in my left arm was the first symptom I experienced. Ironically, as my handwriting became increasingly illegible, working on a keyboard provided a clarity to my writing that had eluded me in my hand-written journals.

Parkinson's also affected my voice. Some days conversation is almost impossible. Coherent, articulate one moment, barely audible the next. Whether through faith, humour or insight, finding my voice, being heard, adding my two cents' worth, is a consistent theme in my writing.

Parkinson's is a physically and emotionally draining disease. Notwithstanding the profile of Parkinson's raised by Michael J. Fox, a future of dependency is now on the horizon. Unlike a diagnosis of heart disease or cancer, my diagnosis was life-altering but not life-threatening.

I read and reread my favourite Psalm 139: *"Lord, you know me. You know my words before I speak."* Aware of the need to communicate before the disease owned me, I began to write.

In developing this collection I have learned to accept both criticism and advice. My experience with Parkinson's has been similar. I have learned to accept help, adjust my expectations and laugh in the face of an uncertain future. For me, it is not only about the journey, it is about telling the story, and I've used pieces of my life, both real and imagined. My stories and poems are tangible, their edges, slightly porous. They cover a range of emotions and frequently hit a nerve. Therein lies the gift.

Parkinson's is all about the breakdown, the disconnect within the central nervous system. But when I hit that nerve with a word or a phrase there is a connection. Writing enables me to strike that nerve.

My mantra comes from a humorous line from the film *Butch Cassidy and the Sundance Kid*. Butch and Sundance are faced with the reality of either being caught and probably hanged, or escaping by jumping off a cliff into a river far below. Butch laughs at the disclosure that Sundance refuses to jump because he can't swim. Butch says, "Don't worry, the fall will kill you."

I don't dwell on what incapacity will look like. I choose instead to write, to jump, and embrace an "abundant life" (John 10:10).

Jocelyn Burgener

NOTES

_____

_____

_____

_____

_____

_____

_____

_____

_____

_____

_____

_____

_____

Jocelyn Burgener

BEING CURIOUS

1. *"Eager to know or learn something"*
2. *"Strange, unusual or unexpected"*

Being curious demands more than asking why. Curiosity does not distinguish between physical and emotional realities. Both are equally risky.

Jocelyn Burgener

NAKED UNDER MY COAT

I am laughing out loud   as I listen, I realize
It's not the story   but the telling.
The loose, unraveling   following thoughts
Endless   connections.
Hundreds   of stories,
Exchanged like homework
Recognized
Connected
In twenty five words
Or less. Can't believe what
Happened I laugh triggering
More random casual connections.
Leading and following. Have to tell
You about the neighbour parking the
Car. It really was funny, sorry about the
Geraniums and the cat. Heard a joke on the
Subway, LOL. Imagine my luck, teacher over
Heard didn't think it was funny told my parents,
Grounded. 2:00 AM rendezvous. Found my neighbour's
pants in the parkade. Naked under my coat, couldn't say
much. Left them at his door anonymous. Laughed all night.

Jocelyn Burgener

INTENT OF THE HEART

When my father read he held each page reverently. Between finger and thumb, pages turned with an exquisite touch. My mother held her cigarette the same way.

Whether bedtime stories, or his favourite "whodunit", my father savoured each page he read. He held the next page as if it were a gift.

My mother created her own fiction. Sitting at the kitchen table, absorbing both solitude and sunrise, her cigarette created a space only she inhabited.

I wonder if my parents ever shared the intimacy of the touch I observed as a child. I wonder if my parents ever knew what I observed.

My parents kicked me out when I was nineteen. I laugh when I tell my friends that they thought I was too wild. I wasn't a model student but I had managed to complete Grade 13 and go to college. I didn't drink or do drugs. I didn't drive and the last bus got me home at 12:20 AM – how wild could I have been?

OK, when I was sixteen, I did take a stepladder on a Toronto Transit bus, at six o'clock in the morning, to Malton, now Pearson, Airport to see the Beatles arrive. It wasn't as if I'd done something wrong. I think secretly my father admired my ingenuity. I had placed the ladder against the fence separating the fans from the tarmac. The ladder held three of my friends on the rungs, one under the frame, a fifth against the bottom rack, and me on the top. With our sign "We love you Beatles" we had hoped to catch their attention. We didn't.

Perhaps I should have told my parents of my plans. How did I know I would make the front page of the Toronto Telegram? "What would the neighbours think?" shouted my mother. My behaviour was disgraceful. I was punished for my failure to respect their standards. Standards I saw as hypocritical, and said so!

The same argument was raised when I was finally told to leave. My parents had been out shopping and my boyfriend had stopped over. My mother was so upset about the family's reputation, their daughter being alone in the house with a boy.

I didn't care about the neighbours, and I wouldn't accept hypocrisy. My mother was adamant that I brought shame on the family. My father stood with my mother. I stood on my own.

Relationships with parents are complex, but my situation wasn't unique. It was the sixties and social upheaval was the norm. Initially I felt betrayed by my father. He had confided in me that he thought my mother was unreasonable, but he couldn't say it to her face.

Fortunately, after I left home, or perhaps because of the circumstances under which I left, I came to understand the notion of capacity. My parents had lived through the depression and the war. My issues were like a foreign language which they were incapable of understanding.

What I did understand was that I was loved. My parents loved me. We may not have communicated well, but by the time I was twenty I had learned to differentiate between behaviour and the intentions of the heart. I questioned many things, but I never questioned my parents' heart.

When my mother became ill, my father asked me to come home. In doing so, I literally and figuratively crossed a threshold. With fresh eyes I was able to see beyond the fights and turbulence of my teenage years and make sense of the dance that was my parents' marriage.

My mother was born in Quebec City in 1915. Her parents were Irish Catholics. She had an older brother and two younger sisters. They traveled back and forth between Ontario and Quebec because of my grandfather's work. My mother went to work to support the family during the depression. She didn't finish high school. When my mother was twenty-three, her mother died. The few pictures I have from that time show a vivacious young woman, with bright eyes and a beautiful smile. She worked as a stenographer for a large insurance company, but taking dictation wasn't her only talent. My mother could play the piano. That was how she met my father.

My father was born in Saskatoon, in 1916, the only child of Elsie and Norman. High Anglican, and newly arrived from England, my grandfather was the Secretary of the Saskatoon Club. My grandmother wore gloves and a corset. She smoked Egyptian cigarettes. My father wore short pants to school. As soon as he graduated from high school he moved to England to continue his studies. He never lived in Saskatoon again.

During the war my father returned to Canada and met my mother at the "Y" where she played. I can't imagine the courtship. They married in December of 1944 and moved to England.

My father loved order. My mother thrived on chaos. My father never raised his voice. My mother was a screamer. It seemed to me that they were terribly mismatched. Eventually I realized they had married the person they wanted to become. Spending a lifetime trying to be someone else isn't healthy. I know because I did the same thing.

I don't know if they came to understand that. Perhaps, had they let me play my Rolling Stones records, they would have understood, "You can't always get what you want, but sometimes you get what you need." I thought I had.

I inherited my father's work ethic and my mother's creativity, but my independence was a shared gift, which manifested itself from an early age. My parents returned to Canada in 1949. We lived in Toronto, just up from St. Joseph's Hospital, where the Queen and King Street streetcar tracks converged. Whatever possessed me, I'll never know, but one afternoon, at the age of four, I walked up my street, crossed the busy intersection, and headed straight into the local drug store, where I pocketed a package of gum.

I must have known I was stealing, because I was conscious of needing to get rid of the evidence before I returned home. I unwrapped the sticks of gum and began chewing as quickly as possible. When I got home, my mother, who may not have noticed my absence, certainly noticed the wrappers deposited at the front door, and the telltale wad of gum in my mouth. I was sent to my room with a phrase I was to hear repeatedly throughout my childhood: "Wait until your father gets home."

To this day, I remember that conversation with my father. Sitting on his lap on the green rocking chair, he explained to me why stealing was wrong. But what I remember most was the thought in my head, that I wasn't going to get a spanking. His gentle voice had persuaded me that the seriousness of my conduct merited a different approach than the usual over-the-knee, back-of-the-hairbrush punishment.

How wrong I was! I distinctly remember thinking I was in the clear when his tone changed. "And now, just in case you ever forget what I've told you, bend over."

It was a life lesson. I remember being confused by the realization that my father, whose gentle hands could brush my hair, and turn the pages of our bedtime stories, could hit me so hard.

I learned my lesson. When I made my first confession, it was the first sin I sought forgiveness for. Had my father been Catholic instead of Anglican, I'm sure he would have sought forgiveness too.

If my father's gift was a lifelong sense of justice, my mother's was the gift of faith. She wasn't the long-suffering type, but she endured more than her share of hardship. My grandmother never forgave my father for marrying a Catholic, and much as she loved her grandchildren, she was embarrassed by the fact that there were five of us. She heaped her scorn on my mother, ignoring the fact that it takes two to tango, and that my mother's dance partner was her son.

Until the day he died, my father honoured his commitment to raise us in the Catholic faith. Even on our summer vacations we packed our dresses for Sunday mass. We prayed the rosary the night of Hurricane Hazel, and had our throats blessed on the feast of St. Blaise. I'm not sure when I started attending daily mass but many a morning I was out the door, even as my father was making his morning coffee and my mother was finishing her first cigarette.

I'm not sure what I prayed for, but maybe faith gave me a place to sort through my hopes and fears. I must have been particularly pious because I was recommended to enter the convent, and in grade eight went on a retreat to consider that possibility. I didn't make the cut. My piety was offset by my willfulness and candour. It seems that too often I challenged authority. It was confusing. Hadn't Jesus criticized the hypocritical Pharisees?

The experience marked the beginning of a turbulent time. At school I was outspoken more than rebellious, which resulted in my share of detentions. I struggled to reconcile authority with power, truth with hypocrisy and justice with control. I'm sure my behaviour contributed to my mother's first heart attack.

Before that our family was normal. At least I thought so. My mother sewed our clothes until we took Home Economics, then my sisters and I sewed our own. My father was a cub leader, managed my brother's minor hockey team, and grew roses. My sisters learned to cook, I learned to iron. Occasionally my mother played the piano.

My mother was faith-filled if not exactly saintly. I'm sure the "Serenity Prayer" was written for her. Over the years she suffered through a number of health issues. My father just suffered. Their life became a fine dance of taking and taking away. I'm not sure who kept score. As a married woman with children of my own, I vowed to avoid that dance, without success.

My parents died within nine months of each other. That was over eighteen years ago. My father died first and it comforted my mother that a suitable Catholic funeral service was held for this reluctant member of the faith. When she died, whatever burden she carried was lifted. Together with my sisters and brothers I mourned their passing. We are closer now than we ever were as children. I miss them, but I have never cried.

A few years ago, while going through my parents' photographs, I received a gift from them. I found two photographs taken at my birth, one of my mother holding me, and another one of her placing me in a box beside her bed.

The third one was of my parents snuggled under a blanket, on the deck of a ship, when they sailed back to Canada in 1949. They were looking at each other, and in their faces I saw for the first time the treasure that awaits us in heaven.

In my faith journey, I have always anticipated heaven. With all its promises, heaven has always meant seeing my mother and father when they first loved each other, before the hardships in life, with its wounds and scars made recognition almost impossible.

In heaven I would see and know, in my parents' eyes, the love they held for each other, the beauty and joy they saw before pain and sickness distorted their vision. The love that was perfect in their eyes, providing a glimpse of the love God has for each of us.

One would think that with my great powers of observation, I could see myself. With my wisdom and insights, I would make better choices, know myself. Accept my scars. Recognize the intent of my own heart.

I haven't as yet, but I am trying.

ABRAHAM LAKE

I remembered my father at Abraham Lake
Campsites rustic, campers hushed around campfires
The sun lingering, not wanting to leave
A party just getting started
My father has been dead for almost twenty years

A child again, my father washes my hair in the lake
Massaging my head, making shampoo bubbles
Throwing me over his shoulder for a rinse
When I was young the lake was never too cold

Pulled off makeshift clothes lines
Rough towels absorbed my shivers
There would always be cocoa
Dusk falls, waves kiss the shoreline
Am I here by chance or did he call me?

SHOE STORY

Let midnight be
damned, I want to
dance. Stylish moves,
flirtatious glance. Boldness
kindled, nothing to lose, savour
the moment, in my favourite shoes.
Through childhood fantasy, anger,
grief, my shoes reflect my life's motif.
The heel, the style, the open toe, have
shaped the life I cherish so. When seasons
pass and shadows fall, fond memories I will
recall, re-live and treasure with smile   sweet,
knowing what was on my feet. Beyond   the
glitter and the glam, career, promotion,   and
handsome man, grounded, centered, spirit   new
I walk on air in my favourite shoes. The   End

THE FOREST

There used to be a forest where I played among the trees
Buried treasure in the hollow trunks
Built forts with autumn leaves
A child's imagination has a power all its own
Though the forest is no longer there
That forest was my home

What makes laughter a memory
A winter's day speak truth
How do leaves spell out your destiny
While dancing to the earth
How do you hold the sunlight, the wind or blowing snow
I am imagination to the forest I will go

Never knew that my adventures would linger through the years
That I'd walk those paths a thousand times
Facing down my fears
My imagination searched to find a home
For the fragile place I call my life
And a peace I'd never known

The trees I climb will call my name
The pond will know my face
Every secret rendezvous will know a hidden place
My imagination is a treasure all its own
Though the forest is no longer there
The forest is my home

AND YOUR MAIDEN NAME WAS

How odd that my name belongs to a security system. Actually it's not my real name, it's my mother's name. To be specific, it's her maiden name that secures access to my account. Is it me, or did someone

```
┌─────────────────────────┐
│                         │
│      PASSWORD           │
│                         │
└─────────────────────────┘
```

turn the notion of security on its head. As if by invoking her maiden name my money would have the protection I knew as a child. It strikes me as ironic, for her name has no currency, if valued at all. Seldom spoken or referenced, withdrawn, to be legally recognized as wife and mother. I am disturbed by the notion that my bank requires me to surrender the very name which forever protects all I treasure.

THE POTTER

She spoke with conviction
There is nothing wrong with me
Neither arrogant nor confrontational
It came from the certainty of
Working with clay
From touching
What has yet
To be
Formed
From seeing
What has
Yet to be created
From knowing what is possible

NEWTON'S THREE LAWS OF MOTION

Newton is underrated
Gravity pulls in more directions
Than a falling apple

#1

Fear weighing heavily upon my heart
Tangible yet occupying no space
I resist but can't move

#2

Knowledge exchanged for pride
As temptation accelerates
The masses are forced out of the garden

#3

Whether self-inflicted or unexpected
The heart endures
Words that sever, wound, bind and heal

NOTES

_____

_____

_____

_____

_____

_____

_____

_____

_____

_____

_____

_____

_____

Jocelyn Burgener

JOURNEY

1. *"An act or instance of traveling from one place to another"*
2. *"Something suggesting travel or passage from one place to another"*

A journey may not be about the destination but it still requires a first step, and a sense of direction. Knowing where you've been gives purpose to arriving, even when wandering lost.

Jocelyn Burgener

THE BAGGAGE TAG

I keep the baggage tag in a tray beside my bed. Sometimes it serves as a bookmarker, but unlike the usual clutter of a night table, the blue baggage tag holds a memory of my heart.

I remember saving it in my passport when I returned home. I put it in my paper tray with my crossword pens and notepads, and at night when I reach to turn out the light, it is often the last thing I see. For a few moments I close my eyes and remember.

I remember imagining that I am hanging upside down, held to the earth by some obscure force of gravity. Swimming through crested waves, my world is upside down, but somehow I am held fast, not with a net but with an embrace so powerful I am bonded to the sea and the shore. When I look up I am among the stars, which define a shoreline that dissolves over the horizon. The memory is exquisite.

The tag is not high-tech. It has no barcode. It is a simple cardboard card about the size of a chocolate bar. There is a hole at one end to which you can fasten a string, but no one does. There is a place for the flight number, but it is blank. HVB, the airport's international call letters, identify Hervey Bay, Queensland, Australia, which is where I am flying from. Where I am flying to is also printed.

LADY ELLIOT ISLAND ECO RESORT

HVB

FLT _____

Name _____ Burgener _____

Room No. _____ Eco hut 6 _____

Across the top reads: LADY ELLIOT ISLAND ECO RESORT, and below that where it reads "Name," someone has written: "Burgener," and below that next to "Room No." it reads "Eco Hut 6." I am on an island on the Great Barrier Reef.

I am only beginning to comprehend why, but like the island's loggerhead turtles, which, after decades, return to the tiny island where they hatched, I understand I am on a journey home. I realize that words are both my pathway and my signposts. It was ever so.

BERCEUSE DE JOCELYN

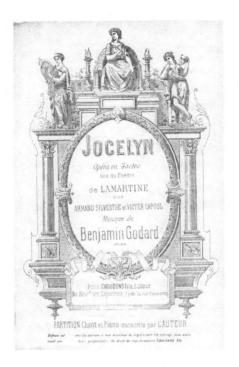

Before I was born, I was a lyric, actually a lullaby. I was named
after the lullaby written by Benjamin Godard, and hummed by
my father.

Berceuse de Jocelyn:

Ah! Wake not yet from thy repose,
A fair dream spirit hovers near thee,
Weaving a web of gold and rose,
Through dream land's happy isles to bear thee!
Sleep, love, it is not yet the dawn,
Angels guard thee, sweet love, till morn!
They guard me still.

OVER SASKATOON

Tonight, as I fly over Saskatoon, the city becomes a beacon
I come from some place. I have some place to go, I am
Almost home

The heavens illuminate towns and villages below
Uncharted earthly constellations, they calm me
Remind me of where I have been
Lead me reluctantly, toward the unknown

On this clear night I see the same stars you see
From my vantage point on the pinnacle of this temple
I see all the kingdoms of the world
It is tempting to imagine their beauty

And stay suspended
Between earth and sky

EL CAMINO

I haven't walked the El Camino
Though I'm enticed by the piety as much as the exercise

I've no sacred journey to exploit
Or convenient miracle to snare my frail heart

I walk Plus 15 bridges through to the parkade
Hardly a pilgrimage towards conversion

Surrounded by executive monks
Preoccupied with capacity and consumption

Logos decorate food courts, replacing icons and stained glass
No quiet pew for solitude or reflection

Still pathways navigated with blind faith
Count for something

Sainthood is rooted
In searching unknown corridors

Avoiding the convenience
Of simply being lost

THE STATUES ON PARLIAMENT HILL

Statues
Bronze, bold, remote
An artificial landscape
Historical footnotes
Symbolic
Episodic
Self-contained replicas
Lost on an illiterate nation
Whose history and destiny
Dreamed or imagined
Remains unknown
Territorial

Detailed well crafted
Artistically executed
Accurate in every aspect
Separate, distinct, disconnected
Reflective of our country

Five Women
Tools and talents
Crafting not a monument
But a nation built for the ages
Seeking neither honour nor recognition
Save a place to celebrate and a voice that endures

(Dedicated to the Famous 5 Foundation)

THE VALEDICTORIAN

I had not seen Donna since our graduation in 1967. Now, forty-four years later, as we gathered for our high school reunion, she was as dynamic and vivacious as I remembered. No wonder she had been chosen valedictorian instead of me.

I never held it against her. I blamed it on the "system", that concentration of politics and hidden agendas, explained away as a necessary evil. It didn't matter that I was left, discouraged, disillusioned and wondering what hit me.

Seeing her brought back fresh memories that hurt with surprising intensity. Though the experience had forever changed me, I knew it hadn't been her fault. The moment our eyes met, she called out to me, arms extended, with a smile that lit up the room. My mind raced to remember what I had planned to say to her, if I ever got the chance.

Our graduating class was quite unique. We had the distinction of being the centennial graduating class of a Catholic girls' school in Toronto. Looking at us now, it was hard to imagine us as giddy young girls, all dressed in generic white gowns, carrying roses in our arms and the future in our hearts.

Now gathered at a country club, we formed groups based on our home rooms, parishes and sports teams. Having found one another, we picked up where we had left off years earlier. We caught up on career choices, marriage, parenthood, and health, renewing friendships in a heartfelt and caring way. Time, instead of being the enemy, covered us like the ashes at Pompeii. It had preserved our memories, and with startling clarity.

This was the fourth reunion we'd held since graduating, and we were closer now than we had ever been. We were bound together by our high school experience, which had given us a common language and an appreciation for the gift of time. We shared almost five decades of living with an intimacy rarely experienced in many relationships.

Our generation was different, as, for the first time, some of us had left school to marry and raise a family, while others had chosen not to have children at all. We celebrated Expo '67, became part of the Vietnam War protest, the sexual revolution, McLuhan's "global village", and the feminist movement. We incubated the ecumenical changes of Vatican II and saw the Leafs win the Stanley Cup.

It was her first reunion and Donna was like a magnet, drawing people to her with familiarity and grace. Four decades later, we still knew her. She had been prominent in our high school theatre productions, playing Nanki-Poo in *The Mikado* and Laura in *The Glass Menagerie*. I studied theatre arts after high school, and recognized that Donna had not lost her sense of drama. Our embrace was heartfelt and genuine.

"You should have been class valedictorian. I didn't deserve to win," she said with a candour that surprised me. "After all these years it's time to explain what happened," she insisted.

In June of 1967, at the end of term, a notice had been posted that a competition would be held for the selection of class valedictorian for our fall convocation. Over the summer I wrote my speech. It was a summer of promise and change and I endeavoured to capture that spirit. I acknowledged parents, teachers, God, and the country, but mostly I focused on what we could do and who we could be. We had witnessed assassinations and race riots, but the future held promise, and we as a class were ready to embrace it. I memorized, rehearsed, and rewrote my submission. When, in early September, I walked into the school library, I was prepared, and recited my speech passionately.

Donna spoke next. I was truly surprised when she introduced themes and ideas and delivered, not a speech, but what I would now call a framework, in a flat, somewhat hesitant tone. I was even more surprised when, a few days later, she was chosen to deliver the valedictorian address.

"Donna, it was the system, and I've never held it against you and that is the truth." The words tumbled out of my mouth. But it was true. All through high school there were the chosen ones. Not just the prettier or smarter girls. Hidden under the surface was influence, the old boys' network of families who contributed to the school, trusting the Mother Superior to manage its reputation.

Below that was another level, the need to conform. Individuality was contained. We wore the same uniforms, went to the same churches, and on occasion had crushes on the same boy. We were expected to be teachers or nurses, wives and mothers. What we were not expected to do was criticize or challenge. The worst you could do was question why. I came to understand that, as my speech had questioned why, there was no way that it was going public.

"Donna, it took me years to figure out. From that experience, I began to understand the system, the game. It's never been one I could play, but I understand it." I spoke with conviction.

Telling her this, I crossed off an important item on my mental bucket list. I was thankful to have the opportunity to tell her I understood. She had been selected, she gave a well-polished speech, and we all shared the sentiment of her words.

"But," Donna said, "it wasn't my speech! They wrote a speech and I had to deliver it. You have no idea how hard it was, on such an important occasion, having to deliver words that were not my own." As she poured out her story she recited two phrases she had been obligated to say. "*Thanks Dad* - note the order," she said, "*for the car keys. Thanks Mom for the apple pie.* I almost gagged as I spoke. It was horrible." She paused. "I was used."

For over forty years Donna had lived with the knowledge that she shouldn't have won, and worse still, had given a phony speech. I could feel her relief. Now it was my turn.

"Donna, there's more. You felt used - but so did I," I interrupted.

"How so?" she asked.

"Just before the ceremony, I was asked to give the thank you speech to our guest speaker. An impromptu, think-on-your-feet acknowledgement, on behalf of the entire audience. Ninety seconds to express a sentiment that reflected the appropriate response of the graduating class," I explained. "I have done public speaking since I was in grade school. I've won competitions in Toastmasters, and in my work I am often the go-to person to clarify or wrap up discussion on an issue. My high school graduation remains the only time I felt used." I had been holding that back for years.

My thoughts and ambitions for our graduating class had not been the right profile for our school, but would I please wrap this thing up for them. Starving to be acknowledged for the words I could write, needing to be heard, I had been tossed a bone.

I looked at Donna. We were like two opposite sides of a coin, distinct images, but with the same value. We needed each other to be whole. As the reunion drew to a close, Donna was asked to speak on the experience of being valedictorian. She invited me to the podium and together we told our story. The class of 1967 gave us a standing ovation.

Donna and I said good-bye, knowing we had been given a special opportunity. Our valedictorian experience was never a burden carried patiently for all those years. It was instead like an aching joint that flares up from time to time when the weather turns. We had both been used and our voices had been silenced by the system, a twisted injustice all too common at that time and which continues today.

Years later I am still confronted with my inability to change the system. Perhaps I lack the words, or a voice. Perhaps I lack the appropriate platform from which to speak. Some days I think no one is listening. In recounting the story to a young colleague of mine, she observed that the microphone was a powerful tool. Why had neither of us recognized that fact? Standing at the podium we had followed instructions instead of seizing the moment. It never would have occurred to us to break the rules. In our silence we became part of the system.

A few months ago I attended a conference and heard a woman speak on the impact of "The Silence". She described the void that exists, because for over six thousand years, women were systematically excluded from participating in education, medicine, science, religion, and government. Their values and insights went unheard for lack of a voice. It was an inspirational presentation, the perfect theme for a valedictory address to a class of young women. I was inspired to find my voice and write my story.

Donna's speech is in our 1967 high school yearbook. As I have no copy of mine, I wrote a new one, and gave it a title, *The Silence*, to be delivered at our next reunion.

Jocelyn Burgener

THE SILENCE

First the silence, then the audible gasp, then the full realization of

Generations, never knowing all her gifted wisdom. Nothing

Written, no frame of reference. No voice, no structure

No text, no poetry. I ache for all the words

I never heard, for even now my

Language is muted. Can I

Speak and will I be

Understood?

Beyond

Silence

This is

About

literacy.

I tell this story

To those who listen. Can

You grasp what haunts me? We

Mourn the loss of the unborn, ignoring

The loss of the unheard. Listen now for the heart grieves

Whispering a thousand years filtered through the ages. An eternity

Without record, book, statute, paper or ink. The Impact of tear, lullaby,

Terror and fear grief, sorrow, narrative music, love sister, mother, woman.

MAYUMI'S BIRTHDAY

1	2	3	4	5	6	7
		I know today		is your	Birthday	
8	9	10	11	12	13	14
			I don't remember the year		Is that my memory fading	
15	16	17	18	19	20	21
or too much stuff	in my head			trying to keep track	of life, of lives, of living.	
22	23	24	25	26	27	28
	Numbers should	only count		when you're on a	budget, or gambling, or both	
29	30	31	1	2	3	4
Life is like that.	You risk all or nothing,		Trying to find the balance		that only comes	with age.

CARRYING OPPORTUNITY

I'm so tired of being wise
Carrying opportunity
Interpreting the reality released
When the Almighty exhales

So tired of conclusions
Carrying opportunity
Whole without a centre
Inertia false perfection

So tired of being wise
Carrying opportunity
Resist answering the inevitable questions
Turn my wheelbarrow upside down

MISPLACED NEEDS

When something is misplaced is it lost?
I misplaced my needs
Spent countless hours
Trying to find them
When I finally did
Realized I'd lost everything

I searched and searched
Incapable of recognizing them
Acquired a host of substitutes,
Sweet talkers, deep thinkers
Who took what they needed

Turned myself inside out
Examining the how and the where
No surprise I couldn't find them
No map, no access or entry,
Doors locked and barred
Hidden, concealed, erased

Searched to no avail, when suddenly, I tripped
Landed unceremoniously, not a shred of dignity
Bruised, bloodied and scarred, I began to laugh
At my stupid, misguided, misplaced footsteps
Eyes looking down, ignoring the path that lay ahead

THE FALL

The conversations were more intimate than the sex. I missed them both. We had met at the Vintage Chophouse, at a farewell gathering for a mutual friend. There was an empty chair between us. He asked me how I knew Paul, and as I was answering he interrupted me.

"I can't hear you," he said.

I raised my voice, but again he insisted that he couldn't hear me.

"Move closer." He pulled back the empty chair. I sat down and began again to answer his question, but he wasn't listening. "I can't believe you'd fall for that line." He was smiling.

We talked about our jobs, families, and favourite books. At last somebody appreciated the complexity of my current favourite author, Len Deighton.

"He interrupts the conversation to describe the furniture, or a painting. You feel like you're holding your breath until the dialogue continues," I offered.

"What gets me is how that process adds layers to Samson's *modus operandi*. It's like watching Daniel Craig as opposed to Roger Moore's 007. Same gestures, even the same words, totally different effect," he said.

"Exactly!" I interjected. "In some ways the characters are more complex than the plot."

The bartender stopped interrupting. Moving together as if sharing a straw, we had hardly touched our wine. We drew closer, engaged in a verbal dance, with subtle movements, and an unfamiliar etiquette. Was I leading or following? Should I have touched his arm, let him kiss me goodnight, agree to see him again? Driving home I knew I had crossed over to a forbidden place. I had not only fallen for his line, I had fallen in love.

He travelled a lot, and his job very demanding. I may have been second fiddle, but when the orchestra played I couldn't get enough of the music. He taught me how to read the score, conduct, and improvise. When he was transferred to the Middle East the lessons ended. He wasn't interested in a long-distance relationship. My friends said he was selfish, a user. I didn't say anything.

I hadn't seen him in four years. Every now and then something triggered a memory, and I missed him. When it's over it's over, I told myself. Still I missed him. I avoided the Vintage, couldn't imagine facing that bartender. I began to write poetry, and although I knew every sentence in Deighton's trilogies, I couldn't bring myself to finish his final novel *Charity*. I didn't want to know how it ended.

I had just finished my bath when the phone rang. Wrapping my robe around my suddenly raw old wounds, I had poured myself a glass of wine, as if to shield myself from new ones.

"Hello." There was a pause.

"Hi." His voice sounded more like a sigh than a greeting. I heard myself breathing back.

"Hi." Then, "How are you? Where are you?"

"Go out onto your terrace." It was somewhere between a command and a request. I went to the patio and stepped out into the night.

"Hi again," his voice came through the night air. Less than fifty feet away, he waved. "Come over." He called out the suite number.

Afraid I'd change my mind, or worse, that he would call and withdraw his invitation, I threw on my jeans. From my lingerie drawer, I pulled out a red teddy. He once told me that he had imagined me wearing one. That was ages ago. Grabbing my keys, the bottle of wine, a splash of perfume, was I really running? When I stepped out of the elevator, he was standing in the hallway, the door open behind him.

"What are you doing here?" I blurted out in disbelief.

"Nice way to say hello," he teased.

"Sorry." Why did I feel defensive? I held out the bottle of wine. "Peace. How about why are you here?" I followed him to the kitchen.

"I'm on an assignment for three months." He opened a cupboard and placed two glasses on the counter. "The company arranged this corporate suite. I arrived this morning, still waiting for my luggage. Thanks for the wine. Cheers!"

"So it was you in the parkade this morning," I interrupted. Was that what had triggered all those memories? "This is unreal," I exclaimed as I walked out onto the terrace and looked over at my condo. I walked back inside and picked up my wine glass. I was going to propose a toast, but he spoke first.

"As you can see, not all the furniture has arrived, so we can sit here or there." Lifting his glass he pointed to the bedroom.

"I can't hear you," I said softly. With no hesitation I moved towards the open bedroom doorway.

I tried to say how I had missed him, when his lips closed over mine. His kisses searched my mouth and I was aware of the sounds in my throat being swallowed whole. Like a kid working to salvage every drip of a melting ice cream cone we licked and sucked urgently. Devouring, savouring delicious flavours, until there was nothing left but contentment and sticky fingers.

His schedule was erratic, so my life revolved around it. Conversations were saved for Saturday and they could take all morning. One moment it would be personal. "You should apply for that position. You know the people, and you've got the skills," he would encourage me. The next could be global. "Malcolm Gladwell's 10,000 hours concept is brilliant," he'd observe.

"Until you apply it to the Leafs!" I laughed.

I spoke with a new confidence, offering opinions, desperate to be considered by someone who thought the world was worth saving. He said that if India and China were the future, his money was on India - yoga was more than a fad. Like Paul Simon's lyrics we connected "incidents and accidents, hints and allegations." We explored each other's thoughts with the same intensity we had used our bodies.

"I'm away for a few days on orientation. I'll call you when I get back," he said.

"Sure," I replied. Why did I have this sinking pit in my stomach? When he called a week later, he said the project had been cancelled. He was being transferred. Time to say goodbye. Easy for him, I thought, but then, I hadn't been able to figure out the hello.

He was so good at not caring. He must have taken lessons. His dismissive tone said more about me than it did about him. At first it hurt, then it made me angry. "I can't hear you" became more than a pick up line. It was a challenge to find my own voice.

Unlike the sappy "you complete me" line from the film *Jerry McGuire,* I didn't need someone to listen, to realize I had something to say. Jerry McGuire explained to Dorothy that when they were together it was like having all the necessary parts. I preferred the definition of completed, past tense. *"Concluded; brought an end to."*

I've used his line a few times at clubs and parties and chuckle whenever someone falls for it, and I did finish Deighton's final book. That felt good.

THE MODIGLIANI EXHIBITION

I went to see the Modigliani Exhibition
I had not been aware he painted in that style

In those sketches there is definition
In his distortion there still exists his truth, his vision
Reality in a unique form of precision and accuracy

My preference has always been landscapes
No, I am not pastoral, my landscapes are prairies
Vast expanses, blending earth and sky

In answer to your question
They convey incredible distances
I journey forever and never arrive
I have always preferred the journey
I am not confident in conclusions
In defining the edges

Pursuing landscapes I avoid arriving
Live beyond horizons, outside of time
Your invitation recognizes the difference
Between borders and boundaries
You challenged me to define my edges

Jocelyn Burgener

MERLIN'S JOURNEY

Travel with me
To a place in my heart
Familiar as friendship
Hand in hand, secrets shared
Laughing spontaneously

Enter through the Looking Glass
The Rabbit Hole, the Wardrobe
Never Never Land
On the count of three

Replace memory with joy
Discover glee
Dash eagerly towards childhood

Unburdened, innocent, without guile
Trusting imagination, heroic, loyal
Willing to dare, brave comrades

Journey backwards
Where hurt is kissed away, scars superficial
Pain only a slow remembering, not self-inflicted

Neither gravity nor age contain me
I am propelled, urgent as labour
To know my first breath

NOTES

FEARFUL

1. *"Feeling fear"*
2. *"Showing or caused by fear"*

Fear is a tangible reality, hidden within our choices and decisions, behind what is seen and unseen. Living in fear should not be confused with living.

Jocelyn Burgener

THE TOUCH

I had said yes
And in an instant
There was a touch I did not want to know
A hand which presumed a place
I had not spoken of
Mine to give
But not yours to take
Now the hands are everywhere
And it matters not whether I say yes or no

IRONY

In a world where measurement is an art form
We succeed or fail by milliseconds
The very fact that one can endure more
Is a victory

In a world where half-truths
Create more controversy than half-seconds
Trust severed
Changes the game

In a world where a moment trumps
A moment of truth
With the twist of a bladeless knife
A second counts for nothing, and everything

HIPS

I am lying on the floor
Hands on my hips
Lifting my feet into the air
Stretching my toes over my head

Precise choreography
I know my fear
Who will hold me
When I cannot move

I am lying with you
Your hands on my hips
You lift me, stretch me
My body moves with you

I know my fear
If not you
Who will hold me
When I cannot move

BREAKFAST IN THE GARDEN OF EDEN

I ate breakfast in the Garden of Eden
Sun rising, exquisite light of day
Luscious styrofoam grapes
Dangle in bunches from plastic vines

Seduced by the irresistible smell of coffee
Misplaced willpower resisting fruit
Order Eggs Benedict sip my coffee
Discreetly observe good and evil
At play in the garden

In the corner
Lovers speak-read the Gazette
Morning news shared intimately
Swallowed whole with a kiss
Editorials interrupted, digested in pieces

By the window
Daylight emits no warmth
Hands fondle knives and spoons
As sunlight interrupts silence
Bruised eyes lock in unspeakable conversation

The cappuccino machine hisses
Coins poured on to the counter
Knowledge begets consequence
I leave the garden, closing the door behind me

THE CABIN PUZZLE

A thousand pieces
Intricately constructed
Carved, cut
Intimately coupled
Joined through
Trial and error

Subtle colour, shade and hue
Nuanced through discerning eyes
Blue imbedded in blue
Sky begets horizon
Horizon begets playground
Carefree child's play

Prized for creating
That which is joined together
Edge pieces
Scrutinized, selected
Careless placement
Releasing havoc

Jocelyn Burgener

GETTING TO NO

MY STORY

He finally left, and soon Kerri was snoring. I couldn't sleep.
From the moment she had brought him into the room I
was awake. They weren't going to do what I thought they
were? I mean with me right there. Oh yes they were. But
this wasn't like the movies where the sex is artfully shot,
and there is a sound track playing in the background. This
was up close, in the next bed, with thigh smacking, heaving
and grunting, way too personal, excuse me! Sex.

As soon as there was a hint of sunrise I dressed, and grabbed
my carry-on. Kerri had brought me a ball cap, but I didn't
take it with me. The emerging sunlight coloured the walls
chocolate brown, making the room, with its delicate wicker
furniture, warm and inviting. I closed the door carefully. I
am definitely not staying, I told myself with conviction.

I walked across the dock and watched the approaching dawn.
The conference centre seemed to absorb the sunrise as I made
my way to the dining room for a cup of coffee. Outside again,
I found one of those picture perfect deck chairs, secluded
enough to send a do not disturb message, and I was definitely
disturbed. My default position was humour. In a way it was
comical and my mind started playing with words. I wrote:

> I thought of their game, sex in the sack
> And remembered the words in
> The Cat in the Hat
> I'm not a prude but that was just rude
> Who was the guy and who really got screwed?

Naked Under My Coat

I do not like the way that they play
If your mother was here what would she say?

I know she would have said something, and it wouldn't
have been humorous. For the first time I realize that I am
angry, and not only with Kerri, I am angry with myself.

Kerri and I were, at best, colleagues, having worked together
on a conference committee. This weekend we were attending
a workshop. It was Friday afternoon when I picked her up. As I
recall, she had mentioned her need to get away from the office. I
am certain she had not mentioned meeting up with a boyfriend.
In fact, she had not mentioned meeting anyone. I would have
remembered if she had told me she needed to get laid.

I don't like confrontation and as I sat sipping my coffee, I
realized that there was little hope of avoiding one. We had
booked the conference rate for double occupancy, not triple.
It wasn't like a college dorm where you'd help your sorority
sister beat curfew, or sneak a boy out of the dorm. That came
with house rules, like advance notice, reciprocity, beer.

This incident was downright rude. Yet, I had lain
there, silent and still, while they banged away.
Feigning sleep, increasingly angry. Angrier still.

I made my way to the dining hall and located a table
directly between the two entrances. Besides watching
for her, I was looking for a man whose name I recognized
in the conference material. If it was the same person,
he was a classmate I had known in high school, the big
shoulder to cry on kind of friend, and I felt like crying.

In my final year of high school Mark was the only person able
to persuade me to skip a class. He had encouraged me assert
myself. To recognize that the six-day war between Israel and

Egypt was worth paying attention to, regardless of the conse-
quences. We skipped geography and went to a coffee shop to
watch the news. He was right. How ironic that almost a half a
century later I was still dealing with my inability to assert myself.

I was thrilled to see him walk through the door. Instantly
recognizing me, he came straight away to my table,
arms stretched out delivering the warmest of hugs.

"Look at you," he said, "you have the same beauti-
ful smile I remember. What a surprise!"

"You have the same long fingers. Did you ever learn to
play guitar?" I asked. He had been a diligent student,
but the instrument had always been a challenge.

"No," he said, with notable regret.

We spent half an hour tucked away with our coffee, filling
in the blanks, when out of the blue he asked me what
was wrong. It didn't take long to share my story.

"So you're anxious about confronting her?" He had majored in
psychology. "Why? You have every reason to be offended."

"I know," I said. Then, in a voice so quiet he asked
me to repeat myself, I said, "I can't say no. I can't
stand up for myself, can't assert myself."

He stood up and gave me a hug.

"Go and book into a single room. We can talk over
dinner. Think about what you've just said, and in case
you run into her, practice saying no," he smiled.

I checked the agenda, and waited in my car until the session she was moderating started. I returned to the room, checked to see if she had left a note, some explanation or apology. She hadn't. At the reception I left a note for Mark:

> *Sorry to have bailed, I was just getting more and more upset. Will take your advice on embedding NO in my vocabulary.*

and checked out.

She called several times, but I never responded. Thank goodness for call display. But I knew I would eventually have to confront her. Actually I knew I had to confront myself. I sought some professional support, and when I was ready I took her call. My voice was calm as I told her she had made a serious error in judgment. Then, just as I had practiced, after telling her never to call me again, I hung up. Then I called Mark.

"It was my first real no," I said. "It's amazing how you can be so altered on the inside with just one word. You really inspired me. Thank you."

"Funny, I have been meaning to call and thank you."

"For what?"

"You inspired me to pick up my guitar and I've learned three chords - G, C, and D - and can play *Blowing in the Wind*."

"Hey, that's great. If you learn the Zombies' *'Tell Her No*,' we can go on tour."

HIS STORY

Kerri told me she had a roommate, but I thought she
meant at her apartment. After six beer and some scotch
(man can that woman drink) I didn't care if her brother was
in the room. Fortunately her roommate was asleep.

I met Kerri at a charity event about eighteen months ago. She is
one tough lady, hard on herself, hard on others and when I saw
her at the reception I had a hard on too. She wasn't asking for
it, but you knew she was definitely looking for it. I watched her
scanning the room. She didn't just meet people, she processed
them. She worked the room testing her mental A–list, finding the
right tidbit of scandal, gossip or dirt. She sought people out on a
need to know basis. If she needed them, she got to know them.

I work with the same list. I write speeches and brief-
ing materials for a public relations firm. I need access
to opinions, trends and players. Kerri runs a success-
ful event planning company. Sometimes we are the
last guys standing at the end of the evening.

About a year ago at an event she was producing, the guest
speaker was my client, and he delivered my speech right on
target. The event was just the right balance between classy and
extravagant. Later when the evening was a wrap, Kerri and I went
to the lounge. After a few too many shooters it was time to leave.

"Say good night Gracie," I said.

"Good night Gracie," she answered.

When she is not being caustic she has a great smile.
Her eyes were sparkling as she leaned over to whisper
into my ear. She invited me up to her hotel room.

We're not a couple. In fact I hadn't seen her for quite a while. Our calendars were often out of sync. It was a last-minute decision to come and hear the speaker. I figured I would stay with Kerri. Sex was always on my "To Do" list.

I didn't think too much about the woman in the other bed. I briefly fantasized that, should she wake up, she might be inclined to join us. But once Kerri wrapped her legs around me, I never gave her another thought. Later I figured things might be a tad awkward in the morning, so I had a quick shower. They were both asleep when I left.

Driving home, as the sun was rising, I thought about my behaviour. Kerri and I were equally selfish, both takers and users. I turned on the radio and caught the end of a "somebody done somebody wrong" song. I was using Kerri and was prepared to expose myself to a stranger, who for all I know could have been filming, not necessarily my good side, for late-night YouTube viewing. Ouch!

Kerri was funny and smart. She was also haughty and demanding. She is the only person I know who can take ten minutes to order a spinach salad. Endless questions. "What type of dressing does that come with?" "Can you serve it on the side? Do you make your own bacon bits? Are the hardboiled eggs warm, room temperature or refrigerated?"

The wine and entrée were equally tedious. I didn't know potatoes could be served in so many ways. She never hesitated to send it back, which I found embarrassing, so I avoided restaurants when we got together. But even at the bar, a simple Bloody Mary took forever.

It's one thing to be particular about a meal, but as I drove home I realized she was equally critical of people. She could name-drop with the best of them, but her verbal assaults were calibrated, targeted and deadly. I asked myself the obvious question, "Who was using whom and why?" I didn't like the answer. "What if her roommate had filmed our activities?" "Was I set up?" I didn't even know her name.

It wasn't an "aha" moment, it was more a reality check. It was time to disassociate myself from her. I ignored her call and deleted her text message. It was time to say no.

HER STORY

I knew she was avoiding me, but I hadn't realized she'd checked out until the end of the workshops on Saturday. I had left Gary a text message to join us for lunch. I thought a joint apology would be the best approach. But neither of them showed up.

"She never gets mad," I had assured him, on the way to our room. "I've seen people rip her apart mostly because they are jealous of her intelligence and good looks. She doesn't argue back. She lets the silence do the fighting." When Gary didn't text me back, I left a voice message, but he didn't return my calls.

Well, I was right about the silence. She wouldn't return my calls or acknowledge the note I had written her. Two weeks later I heard that she had withdrawn from the committee we worked on together. I realized that she was abandoning me. What was it she always quoted from scripture? I looked it up, Matthew 7:1 - "Judge not, that you be not judged." I was angry.

She could have kicked us out, said something, done something, but no, she just retreated into silence, her holier-than-thou go-to position. I poured myself another glass of wine. When she actually took my call, I thought for just a moment that I could apologize. But no, all I got was her rehearsed mantra, "I don't ever want to talk to you again!" Click.

Hardly a conversation! She sounded more like the Wicked Witch of the West, but she forgot to claim my little dog Toto too! Well, my pretty, I have no idea what triggered all this and I no longer care. I hope you find whatever it was you were looking for. Prove whatever it is you need to prove. Whatever you think of me, I am straight up. What you see is what you get. Unlike you, I know myself.

GRIEF

It came out so casually
See hurt and respond with love
You asked me to repeat my words
I could barely hear you

Drunk with hours of grief
Seeking comfort, solace
God knows what else, needing to talk

When you lose blood
Grief takes its place
Wounded, kick in the heart
Beyond sorrow, grief

The bleeding won't stop
Pierced, injured, bruised
Protecting yourself with a flat of familiarity

This grief that comes
When you lose blood
Reflects a love, constant, known

We talk our way back
To a more sober sadness
Healed by hearts that see hurt
Respond with love

PERHAPS

It seemed like a good idea at the time. My niece was getting married at the end of the summer and all my family would be there. A pool party was planned at my sister's the day after the wedding.

It had been six months since I was diagnosed with Parkinson's and I was finally ready to tell someone. Family seemed like a good place to start. Why did I wait half a year before telling anyone? Perhaps, through silence, I was avoiding reality. Perhaps I was trying to shield my children from our new reality.

I remember my first reaction upon leaving the specialist's office. I laughed! Sitting in my car in the parkade, holding a brown envelope labeled "Parkinson's" which, the doctor assured me, would "get me started."

I was recently divorced, had just sold the house and moved into a condo. I thought the worst was over, but it appears that God does have a sense of humour. I wasn't being punished, God doesn't work that way, but He was trying to get my attention.

Over the next few weeks I kept reminding myself that I had Parkinson's. I could accept that my life had changed. It was difficult to accept that, for my children, so had theirs. I researched the disease looking for clues to the how and why. With no family history, how did I "catch" it? I asked myself constantly, "Why me?" and "Why now?" In my mind's eye, I saw my children completing medical family history forms:

Is there a history in your family of the following:

	YES	NO
PARKINSON'S DISEASE	**X**	—

It was time to talk. My children would eventually turn from being carefree into caregivers, as I aged and the disease progressed. Perhaps they would still love me.

Rigidity is one of the symptoms of Parkinson's, and over a period of months my handwriting deteriorated. I worked in public relations and was confident that there was enough technology to enable me to stay employed. But what I had not contemplated was how the inability to write by hand would destroy my ability to pray.

Since 1987 I had practiced a scripture-based morning meditation. My prayer journal was a collaboration with the Holy Spirit and as I wrote, I was able to make sense of my relationship with God.

I have always associated writing in my journals with prayer. I don't know whether or not there is a connection between the production of dopamine and the ability to hear God, but when I could no longer keep my journal, I lost my capacity to pray. Perhaps my children knew something was missing.

Recently, I came across a collection of my schoolwork from 1962, when handwriting was taught as a subject.

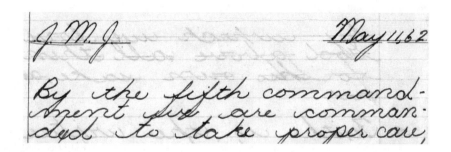

J. M. J.   *May 14, 62*

By the fifth commandment we are commanded to take proper care,

Fifty years later I am attempting to re-learn how to write, copying from the workbook I found. I practice in a coil-bound notebook of graph paper. Because I am left-handed I turn the book upside down so the coils aren't in the way. I try to write every day. Some days it is just a grocery list, sometimes just phone numbers. For a while now I've copied a few verses from the psalm of the day.

Psalm 67   *May 2, 2012*

May God be gracious to us and bless us.

Perhaps I am re-learning how to pray. I know it is not the same as it used to be, but nothing ever is. Perhaps I won't wait to tell my children what I have learned.

MIND GAMES

Privacy

Privacy is not about failure to disclose
It writes its own truth
It holds its own space
Knows its own boundaries
Privacy enables selective disclosure
Defines trust

Fear

Fear is more than not knowing
Fear is about surrendering, about capacity
Not what we can but what we didn't

Scripture says, "Fear not"
Assuming we believe
Society says, "Fear not"
Assuming we can discern

Fear is bearing our portion
Trusting that failure
Is someone else's burden

Evidence

I honestly don't know the truth from the lie
I've pondered every possibility, considered the unspoken
Using omission as strategy, unable to speak, silence is the lie
Though convicted and sentenced, guilt escapes me

NOTES

Jocelyn Burgener

HEARTFELT

1. *"Deeply felt"*

2. *"Very sincere"*

Whether on your sleeve or locked away, where your treasure is there too is your heart.

Jocelyn Burgener

FAMILIAR ENCOUNTERS

A few hours later and I still couldn't place his face. Unfortunately he was long gone and the opportunity to say anything more than thank you was lost.

His face was familiar and I wanted to say, I know you, but as I approached his car I could see he had no clue who I was. He was hesitant, almost reluctant as he stepped out of his car. These days anything could happen at a self serve gas station after dark.

"Could you help me please?" I asked. "I'm trying to put air in my tire. My front left has a slow leak." He gave the pumps a glance as he walked towards me.

"I'm taking it in tomorrow but I didn't want it to be flat in the morning." It made perfect sense to me. Why else would I be standing in the shadows of a gas bar at this hour?

"The air costs fifty cents," he said as he lifted the hose off the rack. I held out my hand, offering him two quarters. His hair was too dark for his age, and he wore it slicked back like John Travolta in Grease. Who are you? I asked myself. I felt certain we had met before.

He popped the coins into the slot and as the machine came to life, I explained that I had managed to unscrew the cap, but I couldn't handle the gauge and the pressure valve. I could physically handle them, but was afraid to. For some reason I felt the need to explain to him that, next to smothering, my biggest fear was a tire exploding in my face.

"That isn't going to happen," he said, as he bent over the tire.

As the machine whistled and hissed, he began pressing his thumb against the tire. His hand moved firmly around the rim. "Should be about thirty-two, thirty-three," he said, checking the gauge. After a few seconds he asked for the cap.

As he stood up I offered to pay him. "Of course not, glad I could help," he said, as he turned and walked towards his car. Other cars were now waiting behind his to use the pumps. I smiled at the drivers I couldn't see, offering my silent apology for their delay. I got into my car and started the engine.

He was just reaching for the nozzle when I glanced in my rear view mirror. I said out loud to nobody, "I do know you!" as I drove away.

I had been on my way home from my yoga class when I stopped at the gas station. I am neither flexible nor coordinated, so when at the beginning of each class, the teacher reminds us to choose an intention for our practice, I usually pray that I'll just get through it. However, this night I was breathing and focused. My mind was centered. This was going to be a good class.

Then, just as we began to chant, a tall man, wearing a denim jacket and jeans, his hair pulled back in a ponytail, walked into the hall and explained that he was lost.

A little intimidated by twenty women sitting in the lotus position, he sounded more like a lost sheep. Again he spoke out, saying he needed directions. Our teacher grabbed her blackberry and asked him if he had GPS. As I was nearest to the door, I went over to help.

It took a few minutes to locate the address, but I could sense that the directions weren't clear. I explained that I had an actual map in my car that might be more helpful. I sympathized with him.

"I am always getting lost," I said. It was a cold winter's night. The sky was clear and the stars shone with a clarity that eluded us. I pulled out my city map, and looked up the address in the index.

His mother had just moved into new a seniors' residence, he explained.

"We live in Medicine Hat," he told me. "My father died last month and my mother can't care for herself." His sister had arranged the move and this was his first visit. "I don't know if we made the right decision," he said. He studied the map. In spite of having received the directions, he was not exactly sure where he was going. It was obvious that following directions wasn't the only thing he wasn't sure about.

"My family lives down east and we recently had to relocate my mother when my dad died," I told him. "I felt the move was the beginning of the end of her life."

Without hesitation, he said, "That's exactly what Mom said. I'm trying to be there for her, but I'm not exactly sure where there is."

I tried to be funny.

"Well today's your lucky day because for once you actually can get there from here." He smiled.

"Take my map," I said.

"Are you sure?" he asked.

"Please," I said, "I know what it feels like to be lost." As I handed him the map, he offered to pay for it. "Of course not," I said. "Glad I could help."

I smiled at his wife as he walked back to the car.

"Thank you," he said.

I watched him drive away, then returned to my class. I realized that although I didn't know his name, there was something familiar about him. I felt I knew him.

What an unusual evening, I thought. Tonight I had asked for help from, and offered help to, total strangers. Each encounter revealed a familiarity that was eerie. Later that evening I lay in bed trying to make sense of my encounters with these two strangers. Perhaps need and fear have an aura of familiarity because they are so tangible.

YOU OUGHT NOT

You ought not kiss me on my mouth
I was taught familiarity
Should not be presumed
However tempting

But since you did
I delight not in the kiss
But the freedom
To kiss with impunity

UNDERSTANDING INTIMACY

When you whisper I can hear you
For in silence you speak the loudest
Within the softness of your breath
In the beating of your heart
Are the moments when you are heard

I know that when you are strong
You are vulnerable
That when you have nothing to risk
You let down your guard
And become intimate

For when you cannot be compromised
You speak from your heart
When you are safe, secure, guarded, protected
And cannot fall
You let me catch you

HEART AGAINST MY MOUTH

Heart against my mouth
A place where my words belong
Where hearing and understanding
Touch

Heart against my mouth
A place where in the briefest moment
Exquisite conversation
Happens

Heart against my mouth
A place where harmony
Is created from past
Confusion

SHED SOME LIGHT

(A SONG WITH NO MUSIC)

Verse 1: The darkness of a lonely night is deeper than the sea
I wander down this empty road nothing comforts me
The why and how you said good bye was anything but kind
Out of the blue, that's it we're through
Just put the past behind

Verse 2: I parked beside the exit ramp and watched as people stared
You had to send a picture home, as if your sister cared
The traffic swarmed around me as I focused on the lens
The photos sent, but your intent
Said this is where we end

Refrain: I've analyzed my horoscope to find a grain of truth
A key, a clue, a tarot card, a fortune teller's proof
Must I lift the moon above the clouds to open heaven's view
And ask the stars to bend their rays
And shed some light on you

Verse 3: I'm at a loss to find the words, don't know what I should say
Did I miss a cue, let you down, was there something else at play
I need to hear it straight this time if somehow I hurt you,
Just spit it out, erase my doubt
Why can't we start anew?

Refrain:

HER EYES

I am drawn to her eyes, they are dancing
Rich in confidence, immeasurable trust
More than joy, they hold promise, excitement, pride, pleasure
They tease, they laugh, they are fixed on you

In that vision I see everything you know
I understand all your truth
I could never betray those eyes
Upon reflection it is clear that your eyes meet hers

For one moment your eyes sought to know me
Held me in your gaze
Watching you, I let you see me

Your eyes saw me vulnerable, raw with pain
Tenderly kissing my tears, with all your strength
Brought me out of my darkness

I emerge from the shadows
Knowing you will never look at me again
Knowing I will never have eyes that see like hers

STOCKLAND CONVERSATION

You clarified the difference between
Who are you and I don't know you
Revealing an insight beyond the obvious
Neither miscommunication nor deception
The apparent transformation
Caught us both by surprise

An invasive conversation
"The distance between potential and talent
Is measured in your commitment to truth"
Delivered with scalpel-like precision
Slicing the marrow of consciousness
Primitive bloodletting, realigning perspective
Creating inevitable scar tissue

Language has the capacity to heal
Whether taken in adultery
Or drawing water from the well
The revelation that wisdom is encountered
When the heart is exposed

THE TELEPHONE

With my "Hello"
You know
That I wait for you

Grab my cell
Watch the call display
Be there for you

I hear myself
Loving you
With my "Hello"

I know you wait
Carefully place the call
Expect, hope, need

I hear you
Loving me
As you breathe
"Hello"

RALPH'S FRIEND

Only you know
What part of your heart
Accompanied him
When he died

Knowing his eyes would sparkle
Eyebrows lift
I get it
Let's do it

If there are pens in heaven
Adding a word
Hearing when no one else listens
Listening still

What we heard today
You have always known
Grief is too inadequate a word
To express all that was lost

He knew the Pharisee's game and the Publican's need
Humble, still choosing a modest chair
And appropriate table
Unlike Abraham, he would offer refreshment

THE SAME DAY

March 23, 1976

If it weren't for the calendar
My expectations might have been different
I know you both, my March babies
By the seasons
Rich in harvest, joyful at Christmas
Longing for spring

March 23, 1978

I know one before the other
But cannot know one without the other
For you are mine
You are me
Your time and space was created
At the same moment I was

SAM BAKER'S SURPRISE

I knew you were on my flight
I watched for you
To surprise you
To say hello
To talk about writing lyrics
To tell you I liked your song
Baseball

Despite the confusion of gate changes
We talked about global issues
Rhetoric, weapons, words
You read my poem
Then told me
You loved my son
The surprise was mine

HOLE IN ONE

I shot my personal best a few weeks ago - a hole in one. Well kind of. Trouble was it was off the tee box at the driving range. Heading, I thought, to the 100 yard marker. Instead I managed to hit myself in the mouth!

There is a logical explanation - you see, the tee box was a little run down. Instead of a solid divider between each practice tee box, a rudimentary barrier built with vertical 2 x 4's was all that separated the golfers. Neglected and warped, the planks created a previously unnoticed edge mid-way along the divider.

With precision and force, and using my last ball, I swung with my aged, rented driver. I hit the ball straight into the divider exactly on the aforementioned edge, thereby redirecting my ball straight back, into my no longer, head down, following through, weight shifted, hold that pose, mouth.

In a recent interview Michael J. Fox made the observation that rigidity, one of the most obvious symptoms of Parkinson's, made swinging a golf club problematic. For try as you might the subtleties of weight shift, rotation, extension and follow through are dependent on your body's a ability to move through a natural swing cycle. Regardless of the number of Golf Digest magazines your read, or lessons you take, it's not happening. It's what makes Tiger Woods' influence on athleticism such a game changer. It's why my ball striking is confined to 50 - 60 yards straight ahead. Finish with my shoulder under my chin? Not in this lifetime. Some days I can barely grip my clubs or write down my score.

But I can visualize, it's one thing golfers with Parkinson's can do. Visualization is key element for golfers. Seeing the shot, anticipating the break, knowing where the ball will end up, not focusing on where it will land. Parkinson's medication attempts to replicate the stimulation within the brain, so go ahead and dream of hitting that perfect shot. OUCH!

More in shock than anything else, I felt the smack of my ball. What just happened? Then came the blood. My friend finished his shot as I grabbed some Kleenex from my pocket.

Concentrating on his own shot, my friend missed the whole thing. No surprise, he too wants to play like Tiger. While I practice my swing, he practices ignoring any noise or distraction when driving. His first question was "What happened?" Then hesitantly, before asking if I was all right, he wondered aloud, "How did you do that?"

No broken teeth or scars, just a split upper lip on the inside of my mouth. I'll live to play again. Only in hindsight did I realize the seriousness of the situation. Not the fact that I could have lost an eye, broken a tooth or my nose. No, the most distressing part was the fact that while I can hit the ball with accuracy, I can't power through! Full in the mouth and not even one stitch required!

That night at Stage West, watching the Neil Sedaka Review, I could barely sing "Oh Carol!" I drank my wine through a straw, and thought, how humiliating!

Still love the game.

NOTES

Jocelyn Burgener

PRAYERFUL

1. *"Tending to pray often"*
2. *"Involving prayer"*

Prayer enables a dialogue between the heart, the mind and the soul.   It has its own spiritual literacy.

I LEFT GOD IN THE DRAWER

I left God in the drawer
I didn't have any time to talk
I didn't want to talk
Didn't want Him to hear me
I am ashamed

Embracing the warmth
Of dying embers
Caught between the light
And the energy required to shine

If we are truly human
Are we not by nature frail
Challenged by death
Relying on the spirit
When muscles fail

Are we accountable for vision
When gifted with sight
Or harmony
When singing is as natural
As breathing

If I surrender
Have I not acknowledged my humanity
Is it distorted pride to endeavour

Jocelyn Burgener

THE CLOAK

(A SONG WITH NO MUSIC)

Market, urgent, constant sells
Futile ring cathedral bells
Crowded pathway wander lost
Exchanging coins avoiding cost
No one heard when I spoke
Desperate to touch the hem of your cloak
No one heard when I spoke
Desperate to touch the hem of your cloak

Fiber woven, single thread
Tenuous shelter rest abed
Spinning chaos into calm
Wrap my body soothing balm
Clever punch line ending joke
Desperate to touch the hem of your cloak
Clever punch line ending joke
Desperate to touch the hem of your cloak

Nicodemus, alert and spry
Conceals himself in branches high
Agile swift up high he rose
But I knew not the road they chose
Lost among ordinary folk
Desperate to touch the hem of your cloak
Lost among ordinary folk
Desperate to touch the hem of your cloak

DUE TORRI

I was alone and afraid, trying to find a hotel, whose name I could not remember, in a city I did not know, and worse still, unsure what to expect if I found my way back.

Early evening and Bologna was coming alive. We had been walking through a myriad of arcades that meandered through the city, defining its space. Combining masonry with art and engineering, creating spaces that served as market stalls and classrooms. Sometimes called the living rooms of the city, tonight, filled to overflowing, they became spontaneous gathering places.

We sought a nice place for dinner. Passing students, gypsies, tourists, we moved casually through the crowds. My jet lag disappeared with the setting sun. The atmosphere reminded me of the Exhibition on the last day of summer. With so much to observe I was oblivious to the direction in which we walked.

Lies and deceit triggered the argument in the restaurant.

"It is over. It was wrong," I repeated. "I made a lot of bad choices and I've paid dearly for my infidelity, but it's over, and both of us have to put it in the past."

Our counselor had given us some strategies to assist in rebuilding the trust that was lost. But the specific directive to refrain from persistent interrogation was ignored. Again and again he confronted me as we sat in the restaurant.

"So you lied to me," he said. It was a statement not a question. I began to cry and shout.

"It's always about my lies and my deceit, but you're not blame-less," I yelled like a shrew. When he walked out it was a relief to be alone. Conscious of the stares in the restaurant, I finished my wine, paid the bill, and stepped out into the night.

When I thought about it later, I realized there was nothing spon-taneous about his plan for the evening. Everything had been pre-arranged. The travel agent handled our reservations, rental car and airplane tickets, while he set the agenda. This holiday was not about our marriage, it was about my affair.

The sun had set and it was now dark. The night had become electric. Crowds of people everywhere. Doorways and benches animated with passionate conversations. The arcades now filled to overflowing, boisterous friends caught up in a Times Square, New Year's Eve, countdown to midnight frenzy. As I looked around, I realized I was lost. Searching for something familiar I crossed the street and walked through an arcade, but there was no fountain at the other end, no picturesque square we had commented on earlier.

I turned and crossed to another arcade. The stone walls gave way to a larger, almost gothic like arch, creating the façade for a fashionable department store. I recognized the logo, but didn't recall passing it earlier. Pushed and jostled, I felt the arcades had become a maze, a labyrinth, where every turn brought confu-sion. I circled the block three times before I realized I was going in circles.

I retraced my steps as I retraced our argument. He had copied passages from my journal and confronted me, using my words as his weapon of choice. Reaching into his pocket he pulled out the pages of my heart, meticulously written, as if in copying them he could reconstruct their meaning and purpose. He pointed out the discrepancy between what I had said and what I thought, as if repeating my words gave them authority or made them his. Triumphant he could prove I had lied.

The pages he handed me bore none of the tears, the prayers, the shame, or the hurt, the love lost or the immensity of that loss.

Through layers of fear and shame, he reconstructed a perverse clarity framed by my words. "But that's what you said," he had repeated, denying the emotional vocabulary which infused my writing. He could not grasp that what he quoted with certainty was in fact, my profound confusion.

My steps were aimless. I was completely alone. The crowded streets no longer welcomed me. I found no comfort in my solitude. Crushed against cold walls, edging around columns, the arcades frightened me. In my panic I felt the crowd turning against me. Like the woman taken in adultery, I was at its mercy. Who would cast the first stone? Should I? If I did, was I now without sin? Forgiven?

Finally, the Due Torri became familiar. One more block and I reached the hotel. I had taken the better part of two hours, but he was waiting in the lobby. It had never occurred to me that after leaving the restaurant, he would wait and follow me, but he told me he had.

"Once you arrived at the Due Torri, I went on ahead. I knew you were safe," he said.

Afraid to speak, I wondered what constitutes being safe? As we rode the elevator I said, "I'm sorry," for I truly was. I just wasn't sure what I was sorry for, or to whom the apology applied

LUCIFER

(A SONG WITH NO MUSIC)

Verse 1: Temptation's a weapon of choice
A sly yet powerful voice
To taste, to know, to hear
Seduction caressed by fear
Pleasure dances her subtle tease
Owning the very air that we breathe
Is faith without certainty what we believe
Is chance the only gift we receive

Refrain: Risking, believing I'd never be caught
Misunderstanding the package I bought
Ignoring the lessons long ago taught
Where in my conscience was this battle fought
I need to know what the heart tries to see
Was it Lucifer or was it me
I need to know the heart needs to see
Was it Lucifer or was it me

Verse 2: If temptation means paradise lost
Does theology calculate cost
How do we pay, what is the fine
Whenever your soul crosses the line
We all fall short of glory we're told
Conflicted by the cards that we hold
Who can fathom the hour, the day
If Satan deals every hand that we play

UNCLUTTERED

Oh to be uncluttered, space within space
Where surface is coveted for holding nothing

Oh to be uncluttered, linens folded
As if for one moment I could be prepared

Stuff confines me, hopelessly bound
Not to what I possess, but what possesses me

BASKET OF ANGELS

Why did I I buy you a basket of Angels
Angels grasp eternity, safeguard us
Whisper in our dreams, speak truth
I think about those things

Angels remind me of treasured times
Of Christmases shared
They call me to be the child I was
I think about those things

Angels awaken my soul's imaginings
Shaping the clouds on a summer afternoon
They breathe the silence of snow
I think about those things

Across time, Angels carry the prayers
Written in my heart
They lay my grief at the gates of heaven
I think about those things

Why did I buy you a basket of Angels
They wanted you to know
I think about those things

I'VE BEEN WATCHING YOU

(40TH WEDDING ANNIVERSARY CELEBRATION)

I've been watching you share space
Close the door when you need space

Manage time at your own pace
Know what is written on your face

Changing lanes when the road race
Interferes with the dreams chased

Thigh touches thigh at the right place
Laughter spontaneous embrace

Dance knowing the same pace
Yours is a love very few taste

I've been watching you share space
Appreciating your gift of grace

THE CRUISE STORIES

In 2009 I accompanied my in-laws Elinor and Jack, both ninety-three, on a three-week cruise through the Panama Canal. One in a wheelchair, the other with a walker, one hard of hearing, the other easing into dementia. We had a lot of fun.

(A) WALK FOR THE CURE

One afternoon on the promenade deck, my sister-in-law Deborah, Jack, Elinor & I ended up strolling the wrong way during the official *Cancer Walk For A Cure.* Our first indication that there could be a problem came from one of the elite participants, who, several metres ahead of the pack, raced past us and casually mentioned that some seventy-five 'walkers' were about to appear astern!

The deck is at best fifteen feet across, with deck chairs and lifeboats situated strategically both port and starboard. As luck would have it we were midway round the ship. With Elinor in her wheelchair, escaping through an exit before the crowd descended on us was impossible. We pressed ourselves against the inside window and turned to watch the 'walkers' pass. Sheltered from the sun by the deck overhead, we had ringside seats, and had we had a microphone we could have called the race.

Not certain what all the commotion was about, as the walkers passed with their arms pumping back and forth, Elinor assumed they were waving at her and she began to wave back. It wasn't long before she became the official greeter of the walk. All we needed now were the T-shirts.

But it didn't stop there. We were unable to resume our stroll. The second wave of walkers came into view, and Elinor waved again. All in all they lapped us about a dozen times before the final lap was completed. By then we were on great terms with the crowd. We laughed as they passed and they laughed seeing the joy embedded in each wave and greeting from Elinor. So much for a peaceful stroll!

It occurred to me that sometimes we get so caught up with being purposeful we forget how to laugh, or worse, lose the ability to see the humour in everyday life.

We were on a cruise ship. The very word "cruise" implies a change in the pace of life. Yet close to one hundred people were charging around the ship, in +35 C weather, intent on completing the course. And here was Elinor at age ninety-three, wheelchair-bound, quite content to cheer them on.

Perhaps they felt pity for this old woman. Perhaps they were inspired by their cause. Perhaps they were simply motivated to keep fit and not end up in a wheelchair. Perhaps Elinor thought, how silly racing around a ship - as if it could prevent aging.

(B) LEARNING TO CROCHET

My sister-in-law Deborah and I have a long history and great memories. Eight years younger, she has been like a little sister since we first met in 1967. However, on our twenty-one day cruise through the Panama Canal the roles were reversed. By day, she oversaw the care for her ninety-three-year-old parents and assigned me my tasks and daily responsibilities. We shared clothes, bottles of wine and a little bit of sightseeing. And, by night, Deborah was also my teacher.

At my request I insisted that she teach me how to crochet. Actually I wanted her to "re-teach" me. When I was younger I had started a project. Unfinished I had put it aside. Deborah was gifted with the ability to explain themes and sequences. She was a perfectionist. I packed up my yarn, needles and pattern. Surely with twenty-one days at sea I could finish it.

My crochet work was far from perfect and often in desperation Deborah would find my mistakes, rip out my stitches and help me regroup. Night after night I would work on my granny squares until I perfected my stitches. I was so proud of myself - yarn over (YO), slip stitch (SS), chain (CH)x3, fasten off (FO).

"You're dyslexic!" she exclaimed.

"I am dyslexic," I responded. I kept transposing the pattern, and as if that wasn't problem enough, I couldn't count to save my life. When I sought instruction from my pattern book, it became apparent that left-handed crocheters are in the minority. But I persevered and was finally able to restart my project. It accompanied me to breakfast, the library, afternoon naps and replaced my crosswords as a bedtime diversion.

Needlework was so popular that the ship booked a sewing class and one afternoon I bravely attended. When the ladies in my sewing group commented on my unusual technique, I shared with them that I had Parkinson's.

I was now publicly outed as a *Dyslexic, Left-Handed, Parkinson's-Afflicted Crocheter (DLHPAC)*. I was definitely an oddity in the group, but there was so much compassion, not to mention sympathy. I felt their encouragement to finish what I had started. It was as if I had established my own self-help program.

One afternoon I sat next to a woman who was knitting and after a few minutes she commented,

"You must be the *Dyslexic, Left-Handed, Parkinson's-Afflicted Crocheter*. I so admire your persistence and dedication."

"Thank you," I said. "I'm finishing a baby blanket for my son."

She paused, not wanting to offend me.

"How old is your son?" she asked.

"Thirty-four!" I said.

I explained that I had started to crochet the blanket in North Battleford, Saskatchewan, in 1975, but never finished it. After my son was born, I tried to crochet the squares, but couldn't remember how to start again. I had saved them for thirty-four years and now as I accompanied my ninety-three-year-old in-laws through the Panama Canal I was going to finish it. I laughed even though I'm not sure she saw the humour in the situation. I couldn't remember how to wrap yarn around a needle, even with the manual, samples and a pattern. However, with all the clutter and baggage you accumulate through life, I'd still remembered where I'd kept the squares, the yarn and crochet hook for thirty-four years. I gave it to him at Christmas.

(C) CONVERSATION WITH A BUTTON

The button is not a metaphor, it is real and so was my conversation. It went something like this:

"Is this a contest?" I ask. "I know if I win I can continue getting dressed. If you win, you get to stay on your hanger. If you're lucky the chances of me throwing you on the floor and then spending a weekend in my laundry basket are very real." I laugh.

Then I move to rational. I'm not mathematically inclined but I do know that if I can get 75% of the button into the buttonhole I have a chance of actually getting dressed. I explain to the button that I am at least 60% through the buttonhole, but stymied!

I laugh again. If I were investing in new technologies would I put my money on the button or the zipper? No contest, zipper. Simple, grip and pull. Although with a zipper, you have to factor in the behind-the-back, hand-eye coordination aspect. On the cruise we had occasion to dress for dinner and I had planned on wearing this blouse. So I regroup and review my approach.

Have you ever noticed whether your buttonholes are horizontal or vertical? (They are vertical.) Given that buttons are usually round, it should be quite simple to stretch the hole open and slide the button through. I'm up for the task, but no progress.

If I stretch the buttonhole left and insert the button on the same plane, we should have contact. Button firmly gripped in my left hand, buttonhole in my right. If clothes came with instructions I'm sure they would read: *To assemble, insert button(s) into slot 'A' - see diagram*. They might even come with a modified Allen key in IKEA packaging.

I tell my hand to switch tasks and pull the buttonhole over the button. Physics works against me. It's as if buttons have an inherent protocol when fastening. They go INTO the buttonhole, the buttonhole does not go OVER them. Pardon me, I forgot.

It must be about the angle of approach – straight line versus round button. Like vending machines, laundromats, public telephones, or lockers, the key is all in the angle of approach: insert into slot "A".

The problem is, with Parkinson's my left side is rigid and I am left-handed. Unfortunately, some days flexibility is not an option.

Insert is a word my left hand can't comprehend. Worse still, just like watches, turnstiles and scissors, everything is designed for right-handed people and wouldn't you know it, as luck would have it, my button is right-handed. In fact all my buttons are right-handed.

I laugh, review my options and consider the magnitude of my situation. Dinner is in half an hour. Looking at my blouse and my button, I make a decision! Ok button, I am smarter than you. I choose a sweater. Am I flexible! On my way to dinner I realize I've had a Monty Python conversation with a button. Can't wait for the *Silly Walk*, and laugh again.

THE JIGSAW PUZZLE

Memories are randomly scattered within my heart
Like an old jigsaw puzzle
Worn pieces picked up, examined and sorted
Clusters of colour
Sometimes a face not quite complete
Often a vivid recollection
Saved, stored, now remembered

This puzzle is a woman
The first piece I remember has words
Pig & Whistle Inn
Thatched roof, winter, playing with cousins
Awaiting a new home, sheltered, welcomed
My Mother's sister, my Aunt
Forever connected

Laying the pieces out carefully
Eyes luminous
A smile unable to contain laughter
A voice, actually, the entire percussion section
Warm, engaging, listened for, listened to
Continually reminded, across a lifetime
Of my own

I piece together the wisdom, gently offered
Golf as a metaphor for life
When to trump, be the dummy, do both
Learn to wipe up spilled milk, enjoy football
Make hollandaise sauce, serve dinner for fifty
Welcome guests without expectation
True social grace reflects a generous heart

The background fills, framing memories
Illuminated ships, sailing silently
I am a princess sleeping in a tower
Moving through solitude
To actual gatherings of the clan
Boisterous, celebratory
Spontaneity generated by her laughter
Joyful in the presence of sorrow

Pieces missing still, I step back
Find generosity layered into memory
Recognize integrity, selflessness, humour
In the random placement of the decades
Observe how others are comforted
Enjoying continuous conversation
Uninterrupted even by death

SEDUCTIVE NOTION

I carry very little
Step lightly
Almost eagerly
Can't wait
Won't stop
On my way

Unlike the seasons
Predictable
Even when late
I come and go
Without order
Or sequence

Driven by whim
Pushed by ego
Terribly unfaithful
I dance with the
Seductive notion
Of freedom

ELINOR'S SWEATER

Elinor was my mother-in-law and she wore a brown sweater. Actually it was faun-colored, dappled with a cream-coloured pattern at the sleeves and at the neck. She wore it with comfort, warm like an afternoon nap, reliable like a second cup of tea.

It travelled everywhere. We all have pictures of Grandma on vacation, on the beach, riding a horse, teaching the children how to play bridge. Back when photographs had to be picked up at the drug store. When film came in rolls of 24 or 36 prints. Her sweater always seemed to be in most of the photographs. She died last year at the age of ninety-four. When I think of her, I always picture her in that sweater.

A few weeks ago I realized I have my own go-to sweater. It's coral, with the same cream colour on the sleeves and around the collar. I wear it to yoga, or with my jeans on a quick dash to the grocery store. I think it looks fine. But the other morning I realized I was wearing it over my pajamas as I went downstairs to get the newspaper. It was 6:00 AM, but it made me stop and think of habits, the things we let go, all the changes that come with getting older.

Actually they are more like adjustments, course corrections that keep you on track, especially when you don't even remember that there is a race, or that you are running in circles.

"Where are my glasses?" "Where is the remote?" "What did I have for lunch?" "Did I have lunch?" "Who cares anyway?" Of course I think it's funny, muttering to myself, as if both asking and answering count as a meaningful conversation. But my children take it more seriously and I understand it is how they love me. Somehow, as I let go of old habits, I replace them with Nana

Time. I am able to kick balls, jump in mud puddles and play endless games of Cinderella.

This year I am editing my poetry and short stories for publishing. I have no trouble remembering words and sentences, drafting and redrafting, to get the right phrase or tone. And every now and then when I least expect it, I read or hear something that is clear and evocative. That tells a story, or captures a memory or, like Elinor's sweater, defines you.

I went with a friend to see the new James Bond movie at the Cineplex a while ago. I rarely go there, as the traffic is hectic. But this was the afternoon show, on a Monday. We even went early to get good seats. As we pulled into the parking lot, we were naming the theme song singers, Shirley Bassey, Wings, Carly Simon, and practicing, "Bond, James Bond." We'd have the martini later. Soon we were caught up in the reality of fifty years of 007, the mystique of the character, the Queen's film debut at the Olympics, and all the sleazy, cheesy, moves. The film was great. We loved it.

As we left the theatre we were talking about the gadgets, the original Aston Martin, and the storytelling. It was still daylight and as we walked to my car, we realized something was wrong. The car was sitting by itself, almost boxed in by the surrounding vehicles. The problem was in parking my Jeep, I had managed to place each of the tires in four separate parking spaces, leaving an oasis of space on all sides. "I can't believe I did that," I thought. Then I noticed the paper under my windshield wiper. "Can they give you tickets in a public parking lot?" I wondered. But it wasn't a ticket. It appeared that as the afternoon wore on, more and more people had decided to go to the movies. I had commandeered four parking spaces and in so doing had agitated someone to the point of tearing a piece of paper from a note book, and writing in rather large but sloppy handwriting, a succinct message.

What caught my attention was not the embarrassment of my age, of being so oblivious to the clearly marked white lines, or even the anxiety that some one was so agitated. What caught my attention was the message, the four words, written two inches high. That screamed of frustration, and captured the moment perfectly. A crisp sentence you would have loved to use on an old boss, or at a cocktail party, when there is that moment when everyone is suddenly silent, and the only voice heard is yours. And you nail it!

Without knowing me, this anonymous stranger had revealed my forgetfulness, my "I can't remember where I put that." The, "Mom, I'm so worried about you," reality. Perfect, with four words, they get it right!

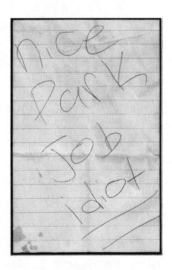

I laughed at my foolishness. When I got home I got some matte boards out and framed it. I took down my Tao De Ching and hung my new mantra on the wall. My daughter wondered why I made such a big deal of the note. She loves me.

I know I'm not an idiot, but the author didn't. Nor did they know if they were dealing with a man or a woman so chose a gender-neutral descriptor, "Idiot." They wouldn't have known I was about to see a specialist who would assess the progress of my disease.

NICE PARKINSON'S JOB IDIOT!

The good news is that my Parkinson's remains at the moderate stage, even after sixteen years. I take yoga for my balance, and am preparing to give up my driver's license. I struggle sometimes to speak. The words are there but the mouth is on a break, so I write.

Elinor would often say life should be lived in moderation. Rest assured, no excessive, over the top, 24/7 disease indulgence for me, everything in moderation, especially Parkinson's!

Shaken but not deterred, I only wear my sweater when I write.

To be continued ....

THE CONVENT

The dentist would call it an over bite. I would call it exquisite. Her kisses had a unique shape and her tongue guided you with familiarity and expectation.

Why was I kissing my math tutor? I really needed to get out of high school. She knew that too, long before I made the connection between sex and long division.

I did graduate but it was touch and go for a while there. To say she left a taste in my mouth would be an understatement. Thirty years later, I still think about her and wonder if she even remembers my name.

In preparing for my vows, I disclosed what my spiritual advisor called, youthful indiscretions. Allowing myself to be manipulated, instead of taking ownership for my life. If my behavior was a sin, I had long been forgiven. As Mother Superior, at least for the next few hours, I was responsible not only for my spiritual well being, but the administration of the school and the Motherhouse as well.

....more to come in 2015

ACKNOWLEDGMENTS

My imagination only goes so far and then I need help. It
came from my father-in-law John Burgener, who at the age
of ninety-six is an inspiration. His late wife Elinor continues
to remind me of who I am and what I am called to be.

In 2005 my friend and author Peter Stockland, reviewed my
poetry and discerned a voice that merited attention. He made
notations on yellow stickies, thoughtfully working his way
through over forty poems. His advice was clear, "You don't
need to tidy everything up. You only have to trust yourself."

Sharon and Rick Barrette, for sharing their marriage,
their cabin in Radium, and golf games. The two
and a half hour drive always cleared my head.

Frances Wright, past Executive Director of the Famous
5 Foundation inspired me with her enthusiasm. She
requested an additional verse for The Statues on
Parliament Hill to honour the Famous 5 as nation builders.
The poem was presented in Calgary in 2011.

Pastor John Van Sloten, of New Hope Church, Calgary,
and his wife Fran encouraged me tell my stories.

Sister Rita Marie McLean, Sisters of St. Joseph, Toronto, my
grade thirteen French teacher, for praying this book into existence.

My colleague Joan Crockatt, former journalist and now MP,
for dragging me to Toast Masters at 6:45 in the morning,
and editing many a draft at Moxie's on Friday afternoons.

Lonnie DeSourcy and my yoga mat-
mates, for being my test market.

My daughter Sam, for her insightful edits and
remarkable application of the "spelling" gene.

My son Matt for explaining the difference
between a line of poetry and a lyric.

My son John who showed me the meaning of tenacity.

My son David for hearing my voice.

Finally, to family and friends, your
encouragement was my catalyst.

ABOUT THE AUTHOR

Jocelyn Burgener was raised in Toronto and is a graduate of Ryerson's Radio and Television Arts programme. She has lived in Calgary since 1976.

She served two terms as a Member of Alberta's Legislative Assembly (1993-2001). Jocelyn led the development of the Protection Against Family Violence Act. Her effort in developing the implementation strategy for this legislation received the Premier's Award of Excellence in 2001.

With a keen interest in policy writing, she co-authored Calgary's civic art policy review in 2003, and in 2005 developed a framework for Calgary's civic sports policy.

She served for over three years as Director of Public Affairs with the Calgary Chamber of Commerce 2003- 2007.

She currently writes for Culinaire, a new food and beverage magazine.

In 2003 she was diagnosed with Parkinson's disease. Jocelyn, enjoys golf and has four adult children. *Naked Under My Coat – Writing Under the Influence of Parkinson's*, a collection of poems and short stories, is her first book.

POETRY INDEX

SHORT STORY INDEX

Printed in Canada